Six Psychiatric Cases for Non-Psychiatrists:

Clinical Vignettes from the Front Lines

Thomas G. Gutheil, MD

Harvard Medical School

INTRODUCTION

Background

In the brief four-week psychiatry clerkship available to some Harvard Medical School students, providing an efficient orientation to the major categories of mental illness was always a primary goal. Since to my bewilderment not every student intended to specialize in psychiatry, it became critically important to present psychiatric cases, not just as attending psychiatrists or their residents might receive them, but also as other doctors—primary care physicians, internists, surgeons, neurologists, OB-GYN practitioners, and the like—might encounter them on the "front lines" in a private office, emergency room, or clinic.

Specifically, it transpired that medical students had difficulty picturing and understanding how patients with major mental illness might present in general medical settings when those patients had arrived there (at least ostensibly) by virtue of general medical complaints—in contrast to the presentations of patients who were diagnostically prejudged to some extent by virtue of their presence on an officially "psychiatric" ward.

The vignettes that make up this book evolved over the course of four decades of my work with medical students on their rotations in the Longwood Psychiatry Program and the Massachusetts Mental Health Center, Boston. Working with actual patients was, as always, a central part of the training—but those patients, in their blessed individuality, failed at times to manifest all of the critical signs and symptoms of their diagnosed conditions. In addition, the opportunity to gauge the treating physician's internal reactions to a given patient was not always available. To fill these lacunae, the "paper patients" described in this book were offered as representatives of those real patients who encounter non-psychiatric physicians in "front line" clinical work.

The "paper physician" encountering these patients in turn was Dr. Hems, symbolizing Dr. H.M.S. (as in Harvard Medical School). For the purpose of these vignettes, what all iterations of Dr. Hems had in common was the experience of having skipped their own psychiatry electives and having slept through the didactic course. As a result, the Dr. Hems avatars (sometimes male, sometimes female) were repeatedly baffled, missed cues right and left, and showed an obtuseness to which the medical students could feel comfortably superior—an attitude contributing to receptivity, demystification, and a non-threatening atmosphere for exploratory discussion.

We devoted one hour every week to the adventures of Dr. Hems. Vignettes were presented in the following weekly sequence: Schizophrenia, Bipolar Disorder, Borderline Personality Disorder, and Psychopathy; vignettes addressing Depression and Obsessive-Compulsive Disorder, developed and employed in a different context, are included here for completeness. In turn, each of our monthly group of three to ten students would read a paragraph of the vignette aloud; this paradigm fostered a natural competitiveness that promoted alertness to other students' renditions. As the instructor, I would intersperse comments and questions as appropriate. Other formats and strategies may be essayed by instructors at other institutions.

Over the decades, some students reported that the vignette approach was more engaging than a simple lecture—or at least, one of *my* simple lectures. Some graduates in practice wrote back years later to describe how patients they encountered in non-psychiatric settings triggered helpful memories of the travails of Dr. Hems. It is in that spirit of engagement and lasting impact that this material is presented.

Practical matters

The six vignettes are presented all of a piece, with superscripts indicating endnotes at various points. Readers might find it best at first to read straight through each vignette; then, on second reading, they can consult the endnotes for individual teaching points. The endnotes represent the kind of commentary that might accompany a "live" student experience. Of course, instructors in other programs may wish to substitute their own commentary, in oral or written form, for the endnotes provided.

In the interests of efficiency, and to avoid confusion with endnotes, individual reference footnotes are not used. Instead, a selection of recommended readings is supplied in the Appendix.

I hope that future medical students and their instructors will find this material to be useful. One observational recommendation for this approach is that, in four decades, no student ever fell asleep while contemplating the adventures of Dr. Hems. Perhaps, among other factors, the awareness that one would at some point be called upon to read aloud was a stimulus to alertness—if not to a full-blown anxiety disorder. Readers wishing to respond or comment may send a note to gutheiltg@cs.com.

Acknowledgements

The author gratefully acknowledges the encouragement and essential editorial assistance of Eric Y. Drogin, JD, PhD; the helpful critical comments of Tatiana L. Gutheil, M.F.A. and Shannon Woolley, EdD; and the countless contributions of generations of medical students to the creation and expansion of these vignettes.

SIX PSYCHIATRIC CASES FOR NON-PSYCHIATRISTS:

Clinical Vignettes from the Front Lines

TABLE OF CONTENTS

Schizophrenia

Standing at the file cabinet, Dr. Hems is making notes on the previous clinic patient when the nurse ushers in Raymond Morse.[1] His eyes on the chart, Dr. Hems gestures vaguely, murmurs "Please have a seat; be right with you,[11] and finishes his note. When he looks up, he immediately becomes conscious of two things. One is that Mr. Morse is a young man in his twenties,[2] somewhat disheveled, somewhat shabbily dressed[3], with a serious look. The other is that the patient is seated at the desk in Dr. Hems' own chair.[4]

Dr. Hems is surprised—this has never happened before, since patients invariably gravitate to the chair *next* to the desk—and perceptibly annoyed. Mentally typing the patient as some sort of anti-establishment, teenage wise guy, Dr. Hems directs him to the customary chair in a voice that sounds a trifle brusque even in his own ears.

Seating matters corrected, Dr. Hems asks: "What brought you to the hospital?"

Mr. Morse replies: "A cab."[5]

Checking his irritation, Dr. Hems clarifies: "No —I mean, what troubles you the most?"

Mr. Morse pauses a moment, and then acknowledges that he needed to come to the clinic for help. He is having trouble with: "You know—that woman and those guys on the job." [6] He then falls silent.

Somewhat disconcerted by this chief complaint, Dr. Hems gathers his thoughts and inquires further into Mr. Morse's present problems. The patient responds at some length this time, and Dr. Hems is increasingly confounded by a number of observations he cannot help making—observations that have nothing to do with the actual content of what the patient is saying.

Mr. Morse sits calmly, somewhat stiffly, and unmoving in his chair.[7] He stares ahead, never meeting the doctor's eyes.[8] His voice is an unremitting, inflectionless monotone that appears to drag itself from his almost motionless lips.[9] Dr. Hems continually finds his own mind wandering into private fantasies—past and future patients, and so on.[10] He finds himself on the verge of dozing,[11] and repeatedly must wrestle his attention back to the patient.[12]

The task of following Mr. Morse's narrative is rendered no easier by the patient's tendency to change subjects, interrupt himself, indulge in flagrant non-sequiturs, and digress continually from the medical matter at hand.[13] As a result, Dr. Hems learns more than he has any wish to know about the patient's job problems,[14] unfeeling parents,[15] abortive military career,[16] and other assorted travails.

Shaking off with effort an almost stuporous numbness, Dr. Hems demands to know what physical medical symptoms the patient has. Mr. Morse responds: "It's the trouble with my cords."[17]

Dr. Hems is torn between his gladness at finally getting somewhere and his confusion about the patient's latest odd assertion.

"Your cords?"

"You know … cords." The patient Mr. Morse glances down at his lap and then looks up again. "The cords to the testicles."[18] Dr. Hems wonders: Spermatic cords? Post hernia operation? How would a layman know about that? Aloud, he asks: "What about your cords?"

"They're sore."

"Painful? Tender?"

Mr. Morse thinks it over. "No, just sore."

Another frustrating five minutes later, Dr. Hems realizes that he will be unable to pry out any more useful description than that monosyllabic complaint.[19] He tries another tack."Have you some idea of how this began?"

"Yeah. It's my next- door neighbor at the rooming house; she puts some kinda radioactive stuff on the toilet seat[20] and then she gimmicks up the TV so that it puts out some rays[21] or something—I don't know—and it makes my cords sore. I know it's her because I can hear her voice on the program sometimes."[22]

The unchanged, deadpan monotone in which this statement is delivered is in stark contrast to Dr. Hems' astonishment at hearing it.[23] He is so nonplussed that he can only stammer out: "Wh-why does she do that?"

Mr. Morse says calmly: "Because she wants to turn me into a homosexual."[24] His tone further implies: "Obviously."

Dr. Hems is dumbfounded; Mr. Morse continues.

"I feel this, like, pulling in the cords. They're sore; sometimes I'll get this sort of pinching feeling in the tip of my penis[25]. That's part of it, too, and it gets me in trouble at work—with my cords being sore and all, that makes me walk funny,[26] and the guys at work see it and think I'm a queer, and I'm not."

Dr. Hems nods mutely.

"See, I know they're talking about me behind my back.[27] They want me to be embarrassed about this … so I figured if you could give me something for the cords, it might help."[28] Mr. Morse falls silent.

Dr. Hems clears his throat. "Ahem. Have you noticed any other—ah—problems?"

The patient thinks a moment.

"No—well—I've been noticing with my bowels, like, they're flattening out.[29]"

"How do you mean?"

"They're flattening out; I noticed that these last two weeks."

Dr. Hems silently wonders if he is hearing about an unsuspected colonic lesion resulting in a change of stool caliber; perhaps that is, in some way, the basis for the strange complaint[30]. He prepares to recommend a full evaluation: "Well, if I were in your shoes—"

He stops. Mr. Morse is in the act of methodically removing his shoes.

"What are you doing?!" Dr. Hems yelps.

The patient looks confused, eyes Dr. Hems, and then regards his own shoes in a puzzled manner[31].

"Put those back on!" Dr. Hems exhorts him. "And before your exam, let's set up an appointment for you to get some x-rays, so that—"

Mr. Morse interrupts, his voice suddenly harsh: "No rays![32]"

Dr. Hems is stymied for the moment, but finally makes his decision.

"All right; but there is another doctor who works with me that I'd like to have you talk to now. Then we can see about taking your problem seriously.[33]"

Looking somewhat relieved, the patient accompanies Dr. Hems to the clinic desk.

Schizophrenia End Notes

1) "Morse" as in Morse code—that is, cryptic forms of communication. "Raymond" or "Ray" as in the rays that factor in a number of delusions, including those appearing later in this vignette.

2) A common time of onset of classical schizophrenia is the adolescent stage; thus patients often initially present when in high school, college, or graduate school.

3) Dishevelment may represent the disorder's disorganization, causing a decline in self-care, including such "activities of daily living" (ADL's) such as grooming and cleanliness. An additional factor may be the way patients with this disorder may not experience themselves as actually living inside their own bodies; some patients do not recognize their own reflections in a mirror. Viewing the matter more broadly, patients may have a problem with "ego boundaries": the awareness of where oneself leaves off and the world begins. One result is the tendency to interpret all inner sensations as coming from outside, a problem that accounts for many symptoms. Shabbiness of dress may stem from the same cause, but may also reflect difficulty in holding jobs long enough to obtain steady income.

4) We would think nothing of entering a totally strange office and yet sitting automatically in the "correct" chair, even while speaking of something else; how are we doing that? We are employing two main principles: generalizing from past experience

(we have been in other offices) and reasoning from environmental cues (the blotter, pen, phone face *that* way; the office owner's chair is more elaborate). But both of these principles require abstract thinking, which is where the impairment occurs in this disorder. Thus, one of the "soft signs" of schizophrenia is a thoroughgoing social ineptness or maladroitness leading to reading a given situation wrongly: the patient with schizophrenia does not get why the joke or behavior is funny. This problem may also be a component of employment difficulties. Such atypical behavior as we see here may be irritating, especially if its origins are not understood.

5) A clear demonstration of the *opposite* of abstract thinking: "concrete" thinking. Such literal mindedness on the part of the patient may lead to misunderstandings. Interviewers should be alert to the fact that metaphors or other stylized figures of speech may not be understood. Basic, simple English is best.

6) This is a classic demonstration of the "ego boundary" problem: Mr. Morse seems not to understand that Dr. Hems *cannot* know to what he refers without context; Mr. Morse seems to operate by: "If I know, you know." Other patients, asked "What is your name?" or "What brings you to the clinic?" may smile blankly and reply: "It's in the chart," a response again conveying "you must know or be reading my mind." The extreme version of this particular symptom is "thought broadcasting": the belief that all one's thoughts are being sent out into the world, so that – when someone asks what's wrong— they must be teasing or making fun, because they have already heard it.

7) This posture, a form of psychomotor slowing, may, at an extreme, represent catatonia, which may constitute a partial or passing symptom in some forms of schizophrenia or

may be the dominant symptom. Mr. Morse has not been treated yet, but some antipsychotics cause stiffness or medication-induced Parkinsonism as "extrapyramidal" symptoms, usually reversible by decreasing or changing medications.

8) Patients may avoid eye contact for a number of reasons: some fear being looked into, as if their thoughts could be seen; others may resist the intimacy of gaze; still others may fear literally being entered through the eye.

9) Flat affect—the damping down of the emotional range of feeling and speech—is a common and important sign of schizophrenia. This sign may resemble the blunted affect seen in depression. Etymologically, the "schiz" in schizophrenia, like the word "schism," conveys that the patient's emotional side (affect) is split off from the cognitive side.

10)   In European psychiatry, this feeling—of disconnection, of inability to understand, and of the mind wandering off—has a specific name, considered part of the diagnostic process with schizophrenia: *praecox-gefühl*, a feeling that arises from the difficulty of figuring out just what sort of person one is talking to. Schizophrenia used to be called "*dementia praecox*" which is Latin for "precocious (adolescent) dementia," as opposed to "*dementia senilis*" which was thought to arise in old age.

11)   The detachment the interviewer feels may express itself in drowsiness.

12)   Listening despite the above-noted detachment may require conscious effort.

13)   These are four ways in which the observer may experience a patient's schizophrenic symptom of "loosening of associations." What is "loose" is the logic of speech: the factors that allow one to predict the end of a sentence when it begins. The listener is struck by the lack of coherence in the patient's statements and the difficulty inherent in following a repeatedly derailed train of thought.

14) Employment problems may result not only from cognitive interference, but also by alienation from and stigmatization by co-workers.

15) This is a primarily genetic disorder, so the parents' "unfeeling" condition may indicate that they too have the disorder or are at least carrying it in their genes; however, it is also possible that this patient's affective impairment may lead to him perceiving his parents inaccurately.

16) The military represents a culture of adolescents, mostly male, who inhabit a rigidly ordered society. Social, cognitive and affective deviance may escape notice in schools, but will show up in stark contrast against the background of the corps. Thus, a high proportion of "first break" (first psychotic episode) patients are detected during military training or service.

17) Again, the lack of ego boundaries leads Mr. Morse to issue a cryptic comment with the apparent assumption that the doctor will understand it without further explanation. A related problem is failure of perspective-taking: the ability to see a situation from another's point of view. An unimpaired patient would realize that the subject has not come up in conversation yet and that more detail would be needed.

18) Concerns focusing on the perineum—where sexual, excretory and similar functions occur—reflect the emotional and symbolic content of that body zone, and frequently arise as delusional symptoms that reference this area.

19) The fixed and stereotyped way the patient describes this symptom, using only the same repeated words, may be a clue that a somatic delusion is involved. Of course, an initial medical workup should still take place.

20)	Again the perineum is the scene of the action, here in excretory form.

21)	Here are the rays to which Mr. Morse's first name is pointing. For centuries, rays have preoccupied patients with schizophrenia; as new rays are discovered or created, they are woven into delusional ideas. Why? The ray symbolizes action at a distance. The sun is up there, heat is felt down here. The flashlight is in my hand, light spot is there on that wall. Some authorities suggest that the ray embodies a sense of "projection": a defensive externalizing of an internal feeling. "It is not that I am filled with rage and hate; it is that they are out to get me."

22)	If the TV is off, the neighbor's voice is an "hallucination"—a sensory event with no real outside occurrence or stimulus. If the TV is on, the voice would instead be an "illusion": a slight distortion of a real event. If the television show is felt to be about the patient, the symptom is called an "idea of reference," where a neutral event (a newscast, say) is believed to refer to the person. All three phenomena reflect problems with ego boundaries.

23)	A distinct lack of perspective-taking is displayed in this offhand, un-cushioned statement, which most persons would view as highly unusual. This is a common event with delusions. In contrast, "obsessions" may well be introduced with: "I know you'll think this is crazy, but …" Such locutions indicate the preservation of insight and perspective.

24)	In paranoid conditions, pseudo-homosexuality may be encountered; this is not about being gay, but is instead a far deeper longing for parental connection, self-interpreted as if ordinarily homosexual. Here, the issue is projected on (attributed to) the neighbor.

25) Patients cut off from their own feelings, as here, might not recognize the situation as sexual arousal *per se*; instead, that normal experience may be perceived as a series of disconnected components, as with this group of asserted symptoms.

26) Delusional notions notwithstanding, an actual tendency toward stiffness of movement is common in these patients, in part because certain antipsychotic medications may also produce this effect.

27) The important notion here is "behind my back": being followed, attacked from the rear, and so on.

28) And here is the crux. This is why Mr. Morse has come to a medical clinic instead of a psychiatric one: he assumes he has a physical ailment.

29) Another excretory symptom: we are unclear what it means in this particular case.

30) Poor Dr. Hems! He persists in groping wildly and implausibly for a physical cause in the midst of this sea of unmistakably mental data. Sadly, a surprising number of physicians turn away from transparently psychiatric presentations and desperately embark on the "million- dollar workup" to avoid dealing with such matters.

31) Here is the danger of using figures of speech with persons who think concretely: they will respond literally.

32) A major threat to the doctor-patient alliance has occurred, because Dr. Hems has not been listening. Mr. Morse's complaint, in essence, is "rays." Dr. Hems' offhand remark about rays suggests that he is in cahoots with the neighbor: they both seem to want to irradiate him. We would say here that Dr. Hems has been "incorporated into the delusion"— a major impediment to the working relationship.

33) Note the appropriate way in which Dr. Hems presents this opportunity: the referred-to doctor "works with me" (you are not being "dumped") and the goal is "taking your problem seriously" (I am listening to you). Psychiatric referral can be tricky business, and the wording employed will greatly influence the ultimate success of the referral.

Bipolar Disorder

Dr. Hems hangs up the phone with a scowl at her wall clock. Ms. Lopresto[1] has never been averse to the sound of her own voice, but lately the flow of her talkativeness has grown to a torrent,[2] and even after an office appointment has been arranged, it has been nearly impossible to get her off the phone.[3] Her head spinning slightly,[4] Dr. Hems observes that her growing annoyance at these calls (which have been occurring with steadily increasing frequency) is now shadowed with a growing concern for her patient.

Casting her mind back, Dr. Hems reaches for that glow of satisfaction she felt when she was first able—by pursuit of the diagnosis with bulldog tenacity—to squint through the kaleidoscope of Ms. Lopresto's polysystem complaints, and have the elusive pattern— *polyarteritis nodosa*—swim at last into her ken[5]. A scant four weeks earlier, the initiation of prednisone therapy had produced results both dramatic and satisfying; results that continue as the dosage has slowly been increased.[6]

Then, about two weeks ago, the calls began. First, questions about the drug, renewed demands, and complaints became established as the usual content of this patient's communications. Then, the quality of the calls began to shift: instead of questions, demands, and complaints came comments, personal advice, and rapturous accounts of current interests and activities, of which there seemed to be a vast number.[7] This patient's usual querulous whine has now been replaced by a pervasive ring of confidence—in fact, now that she thinks of it, Dr. Hems cannot recall hearing such monumental and unmitigated self-assurance in a person's voice before.[8]

At home some hours later, Dr. Hems is jolted from her after-work relaxation by another phone call—this time from *Mr.* Lopresto, whose anxiety comes across clearly in his breathless tone.

"Say, Doc, the wife is—well, she's just not—I think she's in trouble, Doc. Maybe it's that there pregnazone or something, but I wondered—I mean, it's not too late, and we're only four blocks from your house I mean, couldja—wouldja mind coming over and seeing her for yourself?"

It is more to his tone than to his words that Dr. Hems responds by agreement.[9] Mr. Lopresto signs off with:

"Hey, thanks, Doc …and if it's not askin' too much, maybe you could make it sooner rather than later, if you take my meaning."

An unmistakable aura of urgency induces Dr. Hems to cover this four-block trip in record time. Mr. Lopresto admits her, a finger to his lips, and gestures towards the hall, one wall of which, Dr. Hems observes out of the corner of her eye, is freshly painted an incandescent orange[10,10a]. Ms. Lopresto, her back turned, is on the phone, and the sarcasm[11] in her abnormally loud and rapid[12] voice is lashing like a whip. "Whether that's a 'rather expensive order' depends on your idea of ' expensive,' doesn't it, sweetie?[13] And what the hell business is it of yours? Send it over and don't gimme any lip!"[14]

She slams down the phone, spreads wide her arms as though to embrace the horizon, and bellows toward the ceiling:

"Ants! Pygmies! I'm surrounded by pygmies! Moles crawling in the dark!"[15]

She whirls and catches sight of her husband and the doctor. Dr. Hems involuntarily recoils. Though a woman of only average height, Ms. Lopresto seems to fill the hall with her presence, looming and towering over them.[16] She flashes a glare of suspicious fury[17] at her husband— a look that instantly dissolves[18] into a beaming, luminous smile of such candlepower that, despite the circumstances, Dr. Hems feels her lips twitch in infectious response.[19] Ms. Lopresto's manner becomes gracious, even courtly, which renders even more bizarre the unaltered machine-gun staccato of her speech.[20]

"Doctor Hems! How nice to see you, what a treat for tired feet!"[21] She jerks a thumb toward the phone. "That dumb bitch got her tit caught in a wringer[22] just because I ordered thirty silver serving dishes for a few lousy thou!" Her eyes begin to blaze with the fire of the zealot. "It's people—people, that's what counts! We have to love, to greet, to entertain them! What if we have thirty guests, or fifty, or two hundred? I can see it clear as day! I can tell you, Doctor, we've been seduced and corrupted by *things* for too long!" Her voice drops to a croon, as if soothing a worried child[18a]. "We must have faith and trust in our fellow human beings! We are put here on earth to love each other, to give and care without ceasing!"

Though recognizing this tirade for the sanctimonious drivel it is, Dr. Hems is hypnotized, paralyzed, and struck dumb.[23] Only glimpses of Mr. Lopresto's face, saucer-eyed and ashen, and of the two children cowering in terror at the head of the stairs, snap her from her trance.

Two stormy hours later, Ms. Lopresto is on her way to the hospital, and Mr. Lopresto is plying Dr. Hems with coffee by way of gratitude.

"What gets me, Doc, is that it seemed so great at first.[24] She's never been so happy. You know, she's prone to look on the troubled side of things a bit.'[25]

Dr. Hems coughs. "Ahem, yes."

"But then there she was, sunny, bright as a pin, full of energy[26] —y'know, Sunday last, she cleaned the whole house twice from top to bottom.[27] And she" —he colors slightly— "well, she does her duty but, let's face it, in bed she's not exactly a porn star. But this week, I swear, I couldn't keep her off me![28] And it's like she didn't need to sleep, not a wink![29] I tell ya, I'm exhausted! "

Dr. Hems is reassuring. "I think we can set things right as soon as we straighten out the dosage of her medicine. She'll be back to her old self."

Mr. Lopresto's reply is curiously lacking in enthusiasm.

"Yeah, fine, Doc, that's great." His eyes gaze unfocusedly into the distance. "But—I dunno—she sure was happy."[30]

Bipolar Disorder end notes

1) For this patient's name, "Lo" calls to mind "depressed," and "presto" relates to "manic."

2) Rapid, one-sided verbalization, often described as "press of speech" because the other party in the conversation cannot easily interrupt it, is a classic symptom of mania.

3) The problem of disengaging with the patient in a manic state is called "manic viscosity" or "manic adhesiveness," as concerns about separation lead the patient to resist ending the interview or other encounter.

4) Feeling one's head spinning in the encounter with a manic patient is an example of an "observer sign": this is something experienced by the interviewer that has diagnostic significance for the patient being interviewed. One may feel sad or hopeless interviewing the depressed patient; one may feel elevated, amused or revved up by the manic patient. The feelings of one's head spinning when speaking with a manic patient and encountering "flight of ideas" (a continuing rapid shift of topic that can actually be followed) may be distinguished from the lost and confused sensation one experiences when interviewing a patient with schizophrenia and grappling with that patient's loose associations.

5) First, they don't write sentences like that anymore! Second, for illustrative purposes, the present vignette will describe an "exogenously" (externally) caused mania, as

opposed to an "endogenously" (internally) caused one. In this example, the differential for exogenous mania is specifically steroids. Other causes can include—but are not limited to—alcohol, stimulants, hyperthyroidism, frontal lobe masses, syphilis, AIDS, and other forms of dementia, as well as deliria from any number of sources.

6) Increasing dosage leads to increasing symptoms—a clinical clue?

7) Hyperactivity is another manic symptom. In more severe examples, the patient's efforts may be ineffectual and may reflect rapid shifts of interest or attention—for example, when the patient joins a dozen new organizations, but attends none of their meetings.

8) The confidence a manic patient exudes is one reason that the excessive spending or wild schemes may not be challenged by colleagues, banks, or merchants.

9) Since this scene depicts a house call, it should be apparent to all that this is fiction—perhaps even science fiction.

10) 10, 10a) The fact that only one wall was painted captures the rapidly shifting attention span of the manic patient, who shifts to something else before the first job is complete. The color itself is "mood congruent," and similarly, manic attire may be marked by loudness, flamboyance, excess, inappropriateness, and sexually provocative traits. Thus, patients with mania can sometimes be identified from across the room.

11) Mania may involve irritability or outright hostility as well as euphoria. Sarcasm is common, especially directed at what the patient detects as points of embarrassment or vulnerability. Few patients make medical students feel their novice status more keenly

than patients with mania.

12)   In addition to being rapid, speech may be loud, as if the patient were addressing a large audience.

13)   Wild spending is also characteristic; patients may bankrupt their families during a manic phase. How outrageous must the spending be for the salesperson, paid on commission, to protest the expense?

14)   Uncharacteristic and inappropriate verbal crudity or rudeness may be observed in this disinhibited state.

15)   The patient's egocentric vision of everyone else being beneath her is called "manic grandiosity," reflecting an inflated view of self. (A less than imaginative medical student once described this line of the presentation as an example of visual hallucinations). From the manic patient's point of view, no persons are more ant- or mole-like than those that do not buy into the patient's elevated perspective—including friends, relatives, and yes, doctors.

16)   "Manic presence" is a brand of charisma that may make patients appear both larger than life and younger than their stated ages. This observer sign may lead treaters who are actually taller than their patients to have the feeling of looking upward at them. Conversely, depressed patients (as described in a later vignette) may seem shrunken and older than is actually the case.

17)   This display of suspiciousness reflects the notion that paranoid trends and symptoms may be present in mania as well. It is likely that the fury directed at the

husband stems from his having brought the doctor and—by implication—having failed to buy into the manic perspective.

18) 18, 18a) Rapid "lability" (shifting of emotions) is a hallmark of exogenously caused mania. A careful workup to rule out other treatable causes is, of course, still indicated.

19) Although mania may have the effect of entertaining the interviewer, the latter should avoid overt signs of amusement, since that tends to send the patient's mood higher.

20) This is another way to describe the quality of manic speech.

21) This form of rhyming speech in mania is described as a "klang" or "clang" association: an association based on sound rather than meaning (appropriated in a sometimes corrupted fashion from the German *klang*, which rhymes with "bong" rather than "bang"). The patient may create rhymes based upon the interviewer's utterances as well. This phenomenon also captures the distractibility associated with this state.

22) Displayed here again is the uncharacteristic crudity of speech that often accompanies mania.

23) "Hypnotized," "paralyzed," and "struck dumb" represent three additional observer signs for patients who present with mania.

24) Initial manifestations of a manic condition may strike friends and family members as a good thing—the patient is "in a new phase," has "come out of her shell," and has "cheered up." Both patient and family may be slow to grasp that something is wrong

during the early stages. As the mania ramps up, these positive feelings tend to subside when the patient starts to interrupt everyone's sleep.

25)   Mr. Lopresto is hinting that his wife may have had depressive tendencies even before treatment—a situation that may have made her more vulnerable to affective dysregulation.

26)   Increased energy is a symptom commonly observed in mania.

27)   This is classic manic overactivity, reflecting both excessive energy and the lack of a sense of proportion about that energy.

28)   Hypersexuality and sexually preoccupied conversation are commonly observed in mania.

29)   Here we observe not just insomnia, but a decreased *need* for sleep as well; in a manic state, patients can remain wide awake to a degree that would have ordinary persons hallucinating after three days. Such sleeplessness is often followed by a depressive and somnolent "crash" of similar duration.

30)   Both patients and their relatives may miss the "high" of a manic episode – a problem that plays a role in treatment non-compliance. Other than the dangerous lack of self- control and—as laypersons often find surprising—the risk of suicide, "what's so bad about feeling good?" The latter attitude may be a prominent factor in delaying the patient's presentation for treatment.

Obsessive-Compulsive Disorder

When the clinic nurse ushers in Mr. Kent White[1], Dr. Hems regards him keenly. He sees a pale, slender man in his twenties who wears a conservative three-piece suit despite the unusually warm weather. Taking in his patient from immaculate crew-cut to mirror-shine Oxfords[2], Dr. Hems cannot detect any of the usual stigmata of ill-health, save perhaps a certain tightness of the mouth that seems to betray an inner tension.[3] Dr. Hems does observe that Mr. White's hands are held behind him.

"Please sit here, Mr. White. Now, then, what brings you to the clinic?"

As Mr. White takes his seat, his hands emerge from behind his back to administer a fastidious jerk to the razor creases in his trouser legs. A flash of unexpected color draws Dr. Hems' eye, and he bends forward, frowning in concentration. Seeing the doctor's attention fixed on his hands, Mr. White fidgets slightly, then holds them out with the grudgingly compliant attitude of a child undergoing a fingernail inspection.[4]

Dr. Hems's first wild thought is that he is seeing the result of some sort of industrial accident, as though Mr. White had attempted bare-handed to stop a Cuisinart that had run amok. The hands are flaming red, raw -- almost flayed-looking-- with a skin surface that resembles one large abrasion. Closer inspection reveals that it is only the skin, in fact, that is affected; the underlying tissues appear intact.

Mr. White clears his throat. "I was hoping you could give me something; for my hands", he adds, unnecessarily.

"What happened to them?" Dr. Hems asks.

Mr. White blushes faintly and avoids Dr. Hems's eyes. [5]

"They -- uh -- have been getting rather raw -- er -- lately and I wondered if there was any -- uh -- any cream or stuff I could put on them."

Through further inquiry that elicits slow, carefully-considered answers, Dr. Hems learns that the patient's hands are painful but without sensation loss; that this affliction has gone on for about a year but has worsened in the last months; and that Mr. White is a CPA [6] whose work and hobbies involve no known exposure to toxins, allergens, irritants, or infections. A review of systems is essentially negative except for mild constipation. [7]

The press of clinic business leads Dr. Hems, after prescribing a standard emollient, to attempt to reschedule Mr. White for a more open time, a week later. Mr. White hesitates.

"How much will a second visit cost?" [8]

Dr. Hems explains the sliding scale and directs his patient to the billing secretary.

The next week Mr. White's hands are no better -- and perhaps slightly worse. A certain evasiveness in his patient's manner leads Dr. Hems to suspect non-compliance. He decides to press the inquiry in a diplomatic way.

"Tell me how you are using the cream, [9]" Dr. Hems invites.

"Exactly as you directed, Doctor: three times per day," Mr. White replies primly.

"Is it possible you might have missed a dose or two?"

"Certainly not!" Mr. White's tone implies offense. "I followed your instructions to the letter." [10]

"I understand, I'm just checking all the details. How long do you leave the cream on after applying it?"

Mr. White hesitates. "That -- ah -- depends.

He falls silent. After a while Dr. Hems prompts, "Depends on what?"

Mr. White colors slightly and shifts in his chair. "Well --uh — it depends on how soon afterwards -- uh — I wash my hands."

Dr. Hems is puzzled by his patient's obvious distress but elects to ignore it. [11.] Following a hunch, he asks, "How often do you wash your hands? In an average day, let's say?"

Mr. White flushes beet red, in a shocking contrast to his usual monastic pallor.

"Quite a bit," he mumbles.

Sensing pay dirt, Dr. Hems gently but firmly presses on.

"How many actual times is that? The approximate number?"

Mr. White studies his reflection in his shoes.

"Ahem. I -- it could be -- that is, I would guess it might run –uh -- to about –urn -- fifty times -- ah -- or so – sometimes more."

Despite his attempts to appear impassive, Dr. Hems's eyebrows climb.

"But that's an incredible amount ! I'm sure that's not necessary." Belatedly, understanding dawns. "You know, I'll bet that's why your skin is acting up. If you can just cut down on the scrubbing, I'll bet your hands will clear up in no time."[12]

Mr. White nods dully, his expression one of futility mixed with resignation. Dr. Hems senses matters as yet unsaid.

"Why don't you tell me what's the matter?" he asks quietly. Mr. White looks up, his eyes pleading.

"I just -- it's just that I <u>have</u> to wash my hands."

"I don't understand."

"I <u>have</u> to wash them; I can't stop myself. I know this sounds strange but -- I just can't."

Dr. Hems pauses. "Well -- why not? Suppose you didn't wash so often -- what would happen?"

Mr. White stares at the floor, his posture conveying stubborn resolution . [13]

"I can't tell you."

"Why not?"

"Because you'll think I'm crazy."[14]

Dr. Hems draws himself up. "Mr. White, we need to get to the bottom of this. Now, I've been in practice along time, and I've heard a lot of things. I don't think you're crazy. Please tell me about it."

Mr. White eyes Dr. Hems in a weighing manner, then appears to decide.

"All right. I don't know what else to do. I know this is crazy but somehow I've got the idea in my head that -- if I don't wash my hands at certain times -- that -- uh -- something bad will happen."[15]

"Like what?"

"Well -- uh -- I'm afraid" -- Mr. White draws a deep breath -- "that if I don't, my father will die."[16]

He stares downward, then cautiously looks at Dr. Hems, who is poker-faced but non-plussed. There is a brief silence, broken by Dr. Hems.

"Is your father ill in some way?"

Mr. White again averts his gaze.

"Uh -- you see -- that's what's so crazy." He pauses. "My father -- he's been dead for four years."

There is a slightly longer silence.

"It's -- there are certain things I -- that I have to wash after," Mr. White continues. "For example, at work, when I'm doing accounts, I'm all right until I come to a subtraction[17]; then I have to wash my hands three times"[18]

Dr. Hems interrupts : "Why three?"

Mr. White shrugs helplessly. "I don't know. I just have to keep doing it until I have done it three times, then I can stop. Then at home, after I take out the garbage[17a] -- then it's five times for that."

Dr. Hems asks, "Why didn't you come in with this before?"

"I -- wanted to, but I thought you would think I was crazy. It's just that my hands became so painful, I <u>had </u>to come in."

Dr. Hems purses his lips thoughtfully.

"It seems pretty clear to me that your hands won't clear up until we lick this thing. I'm pretty sure you're not crazy, but it does seem as though a psychiatrist could be of help with this. What say I follow you for the skin and I ask a friend of mine to consult on this – unless you have someone in mind?'

Mr. White shakes his head dubiously.

"You don't think a psychiatrist would hospitalize me, do you?" [19]

"I would doubt it; you're functioning OK despite this, but the two of you can talk that over. I'll call over there now and see if the doctor has any time soon."

Mr. White nods, staring ruefully at his hands.

Obsessive Compulsive Disorder (OCD) Endnotes

1) Does the briskness of this name suggest clean and sharp? It is meant to.

2) Meticulousness and orderliness are two of the classic signs of the obsessive-compulsive personality context in which OCD, the actual disorder, may appear; others are stubbornness and stinginess. Note that our grasp of the neurochemistry of this disorder, perhaps involving the basal ganglia or other brain structures, is in its relative infancy. This vignette will focus on the psychological elements.

3) This tension flows from conflict, as will emerge later.

4) Mr. White's initial impulse was to conceal his main symptom, apparently out of the understandable fear that others would perceive its origin as crazy. This insight stands in stark contrast to a delusion, where the patient may not grasp this social view and may simply report the deluded perception.

5) Mr. White is displaying avoidance signs – signs that should be prompting Dr. Hems to explore further at this point.

6) This vocation allows for the application of meticulousness – indeed, Mr. White's clients would prefer it. This trait is "ego-syntonic" – that is, something perceived as a natural, even desirable, part of oneself. As we will soon see, other traits are "ego-alien" – that is, seen as "not me."

7) Psychiatrists adopting a psychodynamic perspective view OCD as belonging to the anal stage of development, where control, even to the point of withholding, is the primary concern. Mr. White's tight mouth and constipation

may both indicate unconscious attempts at such control of impulses.

8) Full-blown miserliness may not be the presenting form of withholding; milder forms, such as marked thrift or heightened cost-consciousness, are often observed.

9) Note here that "tell me how..." is more neutral and less accusing than "are you using it correctly?"

10) Part of the obsessional construct is the perceived need to follow "the letter of the law," at times in conflict with the spirit. This posture may lead to arguments, nit picking and a refusal to compromise.

11) This is so Hems! As implied in the Schizophrenia vignette in this book, "Many physicians would rather be torn apart by wild Caucasian ponies than to admit that a given presentation has a psychiatric component."

12) Realization dawns -- but about the wrong issue.

13) Stubbornness is another classic trait in obsessional states, coupled here with fear of revelation.

14) Fear of being thought crazy, as noted in #4 above, is actually a sign of insight; but it also constitutes a reason to want to hide the content.

15) Here we confront the psychological core of this disorder. In psychodynamic terms, an impulse that is forbidden or conflicted arises from the unconscious; in the conscious mind it takes the form of an obsession or obsessive concern. The compulsion symbolically counters and resists the impulse underlying the obsession. Note that persons with phobia fear harm befalling themselves, while obsessive persons – feeling guilt for their impulses -- fear that harm will befall others. Lord and Lady Macbeth and Pontius Pilate

present classic examples of hand washing as an attempt to expiate guilt.

16)   The father's "death"-- the fantasized outcome of hostile impulses toward the father image inside Mr. White's head -- is the feared harm that has been transformed into an obsessive concern.

17)   17a) Actions symbolizing loss or death, even remotely, may trigger the compulsion.

18)   As symptom presentations evolve, certain compulsive actions may be repeated a specific number of times; over time, multiples of those actions may be "required." The obsessive-compulsive mechanism is neither stable nor totally effective in countering the underlying impulse -- which still threatens to break through – with the result that some compulsions (such as the compulsion to count things) are based purely on numbers.

Depression

Scanning the chart in preparation for her next office appointment with Ms.

Burton[1], Dr . Hems is slightly puzzled as to why she called for the appointment, since her

colitis[2] had seemed well resolved on last check. Recalling that Ms. Burton is a delight to

talk to, regaling her during each examination with witty, non-stop stories that lampoon her

relatives while gently making fun of herself as well,[3] Dr. Hems looks up with brisk

interest as his patient is ushered in by the nurse.

The moment Dr. Hems lays eyes on her, she can barely suppress a start of shock,

as she stares at her long-time patient. Though unquestionably still Ms. Burton, this woman

has been profoundly transformed. Steadying herself by an effort of will and murmuring

the standard pleasantries in a preoccupied way, Dr. Hems peers closely at her patient.

In the four months since Dr. Hems has seen her last, Ms. Burton appears to have aged

twenty years[4], though she is a woman still in middle life[5]. Continuing the inventory, she notes

that, contrary to her usual custom, this patient wears no makeup or perfume[6]; her usual

meticulous[6a] hairdo is in mild dishevelment[6b]; and her brow and eyes are contracted in a wince

of pain, while her sunken lower face appears slack and nerveless around her cracked and dry-

looking lips[7]. Her hand, when shaken, is thin and flaccid, and she eases her body into the chair

with the sighing effort of some one lowering massive weight, although to Dr. Hems's trained

eye, she is clearly much thinner than usual[8]. Unbidden, and unwelcome, the doctor's thoughts

prompt her: "Occult carcinoma, somewhere, " but she brushes this notion aside and injects a totally hypocritical cheer into her voice as she asks: "Well, what can I do for you today?"

At first, Ms. Burton does not appear to hear the question, since her blank gaze does not deviate from a spot somewhere near the center of the carpet[9]. Minutes seem to pass as Dr. Hems fidgets. Finally, the patient shrugs her shoulders, with the manner of Atlas shifting the heavens' weight, and says, almost inaudibly, "Perhaps I shouldn't have come."[10]

Now deeply concerned as well as baffled by her patient's alteration, Dr. Hems presses the inquiry.

"What has been happening with you?"

Another silent pause ensues. Dr. Hems feels her face frowning[11] and consciously rearranges her expression to a more neutral one. Ms. Burton sighs.

"Everything -I don't -- I guess --" a pause -- "It doesn't seem I ever finish."[12] She lapses into silence and stares again at the floor.

Finding herself irritated despite herself at the slow vagueness of her patient's response[11a], Dr. Hems takes hold of herself, sits back in her chair, and tosses the medical chart onto the desk with the quite conscious intent of conveying a readiness to listen.[13] She hopes that this demonstration of openness will somehow break the feeling in the room: that Ms. Burton's words are emerging like pulled teeth.

The maneuver is in vain. Dr. Hems begins to stray into fantasy, loses the thread, and catches herself just at the brink of dozing off[14], as Ms. Burton, with excruciating slowness, responds, one word at a time, in an inflectionless monotone. She slumps in her chair as motionless and expressionless as a clay figurine, without even a flicker of the sprightly gestures with which she usually punctuates her stories.[15]

What Ms. Burton cannot finish, it appears, is the housework. A meticulous, perhaps even over-conscientious housekeeper at most times[16], she finds herself unable to address the simplest task without feeling it to be a burden. The greatest burden is eventually identified as time, which stretches to many times its normal duration[17]. One day drags into the next with little or no distinction.

"I just -- I don't know -- I don't have the energy.["][18]

"Do you get enough sleep?"

There is no answer for many long moments.

Then Ms. Burton's head shakes, barely perceptibly.

"I lie in bed a lot but — not much sleep."[19]

Persistent further questioning elicits the facts that Ms. Burton's joints ache, her mouth is dry, and her "bowels are bound.[20]"

"What are you eating these days?" Dr. Hems asks.

"Enough to live on." She pauses. "Nothing tastes right, anyway[21]; I just don't enjoy eating anymore[22]."

"Is there anything you do enjoy?"

Ms. Burton shrugs again. "I can't think of anything.[22b] I can't --" She pauses again and glances apologetically at Dr. Hems. "I can't even stand for Charlie to -- you know -- touch me[23]. It just hurts and it isn't any good for me. I -- there are -- I hate to say this but --" Her eyes wander to the window, open to the Autumn breeze[24], that looks out over the city, twenty-two stories down[25] -- "there are times when I think I just can't make it.[26]"

A chill courses down Dr. Hems' spine[27] and, though she cannot name her fear, she turns energetically to further questions, with a sense of shaking off a shadow[28].

"How long has this been going on?"

Ms. Burton's eyes, still staring at the window, grow unfocussed as she struggles to recall. "Was it three -or four weeks -- no, I guess it was early September. I remember because Becky was packing up for college."

"Ah, yes, Becky's your youngest, isn't she?"

"Mm. The baby of the family[29]." Ms. Burton's attempted smile is a ghastly spasm[30].

Dr. Hems clears her throat, herself feeling somehow brighter at the prospect of action[31].

"Well, let's check you over and see what's what, and then we can get down to cases and start fixing you up[.32]"

Ms. Burton looks dubiously at Dr. Hems but gets laboriously to her feet as Dr. Hems calls in her assistant.

Depression endnotes

1) Ms. Burton's surname is deliberately chosen. In 1621, the widely read scholar, Robert Burton, wrote a treatise called "The Anatomy of Melancholy" which contained essentially everything written about depression at the time; this was before Google. More importantly, Burton said he wrote it to keep from succumbing to it: a classic example of work as an antidote to depression.

2) Including this condition makes the point that depression can manifest in a myriad of physical symptoms, ranging from bowel disturbances to severe illnesses; contrariwise, many physical conditions can manifest as depression, from headache to Huntington's chorea to pancreatic cancer and others.

3) Ms. Burton's usual display of levity reminds us that humor, especially satire and sarcasm, has always been a defense against depression; as this book is being written, a legendary comedian, Robin Williams, has just committed suicide after struggling with depression for years. Some practitioners recognize an entity called masked depression or "smiling depression" which is self-explanatory, but poses a challenge to diagnosticians.

4) The phrase, "patient appears older than stated age" is commonly featured in medical workups. One of the reasons for this manifestation in mental health is the striking effect of depression on body, face and mind. Conversely, a definitive sign of mania is the fact that the "patient looks years younger than stated age."

5) Mid-life is tough on almost everybody, but menopause poses particular challenges, both physical and mental. Clinicians once spoke of "involutional melancholia," a severe depression that manifested in menopause; it was particularly responsive to electroconvulsive therapy and usually occurred in the context of a pre-existing obsessional

personality disorder or traits such as meticulousness and compulsiveness.

6) 6a, 6b) Ms. Burton has suffered a marked decline in personal self-care (in clinical parlance: ADL's, activities of daily living, including grooming). Depressive apathy is the usual reason, as well as lack of energy. Reference to this patient's previous meticulousness is specifically noted for contrast with her present state.

7) The wince of the upper face and slackness of the lower is referred to as the "depressive facies."

8) Weight loss commonly results from depressive anorexia, but the patient's slowed and stiff movements may appear to be those of a heavier person. Patients who mask their depression by compulsive over-eating will, of course, appear heavier.

9) As part of psychomotor slowing (of mind as well as body), there is increased "response latency": a greater interval between your question and the patient's response.

10)   In concert with the lowered self esteem that accompanies depression, patients may feel undeserving of help, too guilty to ask for it, or that they are wasting the clinician's time.

11)   11a) The clinical response to these patients is occasionally anger or resentment; this may not be expressed or even experienced at first, but one's own involuntary facial expression may be a clue. Experienced clinicians pay attention to their own inner responses to the patient for the diagnostic value that may accrue. The issue represents another aspect of "observer signs." These are treaters' responses that – through empathy and the contagion of human experience -- indirectly illuminate the patient's condition. With depressed patients, sadness, helplessness and hopelessness, as well as irritation, are common observer signs.

12) Not even the sentence. The patient's effort fades easily.

13) The behavior utilized here by Dr. Hems sometimes works, communicating: "Let's just

get down to talking about what really matters." Turning one's back on the electronic health record or computer screen in order to face the patient directly may achieve a similar effect.

14) Paying careful attention to a severely depressed patient, despite its necessity, is no easy matter; it is tiring, uncomfortable, and may represent a strain on the interviewer's personal resources. This reaction may play a role in why front-line, non-psychiatric personnel are eager to transfer the patient elsewhere and why serious depression may be missed.

15) Psychomotor retardation, by definition, slows down both mind and body. Body language may suggest depression by manifesting empty, ineffectual circular gestures; decrease in physical animation in a previously animated conversationalist like Ms. Burton; inability to think of things that should be accessible, and the like.

16) Here we find evidence of some previously manifested obsessional traits, consistent with earlier observations on behavioral precursors of some caaes of depression; see #5 above.

17) For manic patients, time speeds up; for depressed patients, it slows down, often leading to a "stuck" feeling.

18) Loss of energy, or anergia, is a common consequence of depression. A patient may say, "I just can't get started in the morning."

19) Sleep patterns are often affected in three common ways: insomnia and difficulty falling asleep; hypersomnia, or sleeping all the time; or early morning wakening, where the patient wakes in the early morning (i.e., earlier than the routine would require) and cannot fall back to sleep. Awakening without feeling rested is common.

20) Here we find three of the many physical symptoms that may accompany clinical depression.

21) Changes in taste may occur with depression alone, but should alert the physician to possible organic factors as well.

22, 22a, 23) Loss of appetite, loss of pleasure in eating and frank anorexia may occur, occasioning severe weight loss in some cases. This symptom may occur against a backdrop of general anhedonia, the inability to experience pleasure or enjoyment of previously enjoyable activities.

Loss of libido and enjoyment of sexual relations may be accompanied by physical symptoms such as dyspareunia, painful or uncomfortable intercourse.

24) The "Autumn breeze" is another deliberate clue: Autumn and Spring appear to be the peak seasons for mood disorders.

25) We enter a realm of subtlety here. Dr. Hems knows where his office is, of course; but this section of the vignette enters his unconscious, as it were; and he is suddenly aware of the drop outside his window; why might that be?

26) The patient here expresses what is usually termed "passive suicidal ideation": not the active plan to harm or kill oneself, but a helpless sense of not being able to make it, feeling one's time on earth is over, thinking about just not waking up again. This passivity is in no way reassuring nor is it an argument for decreased vigilance, as passive may turn into active suicidal efforts at any point. Families need to be alerted to the association between depression and suicide which clinicians take so much for granted as obvious: after the death the family may say, "We knew our loved one was depressed as hell, but we never imagined he would kill himself." Recruiting the family to be alert for the patient's acquisition of suicidal instruments, giving away one's personal possessions and "putting one's affairs in order" are areas where family observation may be very helpful in preventing a suicide. Telling families to remove firearms from the house is critical.

27) Dr. Hems is ignoring an important observer sign here. Depression makes us feel sad and

hopeless; but latent or unexpressed suicidality may make us feel afraid. Dr. Hems, indeed, feels this but employs a common avoidance maneuver.

28) Action is a remedy for felt helplessness, but action may take many forms. In medical work, getting busy or beginning the "million-dollar workup" are examples, often coupled with ignoring the patient's affective state. Clearly, at her age, Ms. Burton would require some level of medical clearance, but treaters must learn to note avoidance maneuvers in themselves (and in their patients, for that matter).

29) The patient is alluding to the "empty nest syndrome" that parents may experience when the last child leaves the home: moving out, going to college, making extended travel plans and so on. While many parents may feel mixed or sad feelings when the last child leaves, this syndrome may lead to full-fledged depression in vulnerable individuals; perhaps that is happening here.

30) A parent may smile at a child's going to college, but the quality of Ms. Burton's smile may alert the observer to masked depression or "smiling depression" as noted earlier.

31) Feeling yourself cheer up at the prospect of action may throw your own previous empathic depressive response into a clearer light.

32) Just one of those content-free phrases we doctors use at times.

Borderline Personality Disorder

Dr. Hems is on night duty in the emergency room when Lee Smith[1] is brought in by her worried boyfriend; the patient has taken a moderate overdose of Valium.[2] While supportive measures are begun, but before Dr. Hems actually sees Ms. Smith,[3] she is interrupted by four calls in rapid succession concerning that very patient.

The first call is long-distance from the patient's father, a bank president in a distant city[4] who pleads that Dr. Hems have her seen by "a specialist" at any price.[5] The second is from the patient's roommate, who has been "worried sick" about her for several weeks and asks after her condition.[6] The third is from her very upset minister-counselor[7], who becomes so verbally abusive[8] in response to Dr. Hems' non-committal answers that the doctor has to hang up the phone. The fourth is from a local internist who is following the patient for headaches, anxiety and irritable colon.[9] The internist admits to having prescribed the Valium in question and requests—rather to Dr. Hems' annoyance[10]—that pains be taken to treat her with "special care,"[11] and stresses in particular the importance of finding nurses noted for being "very understanding" since, when the patient was at another hospital for elective gall bladder surgery,[12] the nurses there "just didn't work out."[13]

Dr. Hems' ability to attend to these calls is somewhat compromised by the boyfriend's recurrent interruptions. He is ashen-faced, trembling, and clearly near panic.

Dr. Hems finally gets to see her patient—a small, slender, shorthaired, pale young woman in a shirt and jeans[14] who is already sitting up on the stretcher. In a faint voice, she gives her age as 23, although she appears much younger.[15] When queried about her overdose, the patient turns wounded eyes on her boyfriend, raises a tremulous forefinger to point at his equally tremulous form, and quavers, "I did it … because of YOU!"[16]

Looking stricken, the boyfriend blurts: "Don't talk that way! We'll work it out! I'll stay—I won't move out!"[17]

Ms. Smith looks pleadingly at Dr. Hems. "I—just want to be alone."

Immediately, Dr. Hems finds herself[18] gently but firmly ushering the boyfriend out. When she returns, Ms. Smith places a pallid hand on her arm and asks, in a soft and child-like tone: "You'll help me, won't you?"[19]

Quite moved, Dr. Hems answers: "I'll certainly try. Why don't you tell me what's troubling you?"

Dr. Hems' recent postgraduate course in counseling[20] comes readily to mind as Ms. Smith speaks fairly spontaneously of her disappointments with men;[21] her cold, uncaring mother, now hospitalized in a mental institution;[22] her indulgent but preoccupied father;[23] and her high scholastic achievement coupled with a sense of directionlessness.[24]

Dr. Hems finds Ms. Smith appealing, interesting, intelligent, and insightful[25]

… and, at a deeper level, something about this patient's isolation and vulnerability touches a chord in Dr. Hems, whose recent bereavement by her husband's death is certainly still fresh enough to enhance her understanding of loneliness.[26]

Dr. Hems is just noting, with covert astonishment, that an hour and a quarter has zipped by unnoticed, when the patient comments: "You know, I've never told these things

to anyone before.[27] My internist means well, but he's just not as … sensitive as you are.[28]
Couldn't we talk some more?"

Dr. Hems has privately been planning to devote some time—somehow—to the more personal aspects of medicine.[29] In this patient, she sees the place to start. They initially discuss making an appointment for the following week, but Ms. Smith seems so distressed at the prospect of this delay that they set up a meeting during another patient's time. Dr. Hems reasons that the other commitment can easily be rescheduled.[30]

Ms. Smith presents for her first appointment with a crisis centering around her boyfriend—she has discovered he is a drug addict, yet she loves him too much to leave him.[31] At the end of the session, she has some difficulty leaving because "we're just getting to the important part."[32] The thought of a full waiting room gives the resolve to Dr. Hems to stop, but she offers to reschedule an extra appointment at the end of the day.[33]

Dr. Hems finds the sessions rewarding—especially as the patient is so eager and enthusiastic, and communicates so clearly at every turn just how helpful the doctor is being.[34] Dr. Hems is somewhat uncomfortable, however, with the increasingly intense verbal criticism—merging into abuse—that the patient heaps on her internist, who is being berated with near-savage ferocity for faults and slights that strain credulity.[35]

One day, Dr. Hems is forced to postpone Ms. Smith's standing appointment to a later date, and tells her so during the preceding session. An astonishing transformation occurs. The patient, usually waif-like and suppliant, glares at Dr. Hems crimson-faced, and appears to be gathering herself for a scathing denunciation. Dr. Hems hastily alters her appointment plans to return to the status quo, and the patient relaxes dramatically.[36]

As the time goes on, Ms. Smith's crises become more frequent and more dramatic.

Increasingly, her appointments—as many as three in one week—become supplemented by calls after hours. Weekend separations from the doctor seem to engender panic in this patient; boyfriends are now absent from the picture. Most discouraging of all, Ms. Smith, despite Dr. Hems's underlying optimism, is clearly becoming worse—spending large parts of the day sleeping, dropping out of school, and even sounding a trifle bizarre in some of her phone calls, seeming unclear at times who Dr. Hems even is.[37]

During one session Ms. Smith, speaking about her intense anxiety, is obviously beginning to feel it in the room. Suddenly, she stares at Dr. Hems and cries: "Aah! Your face is melting!"[38]

Dr. Hems is startled and draws back in her chair. The patient rubs her eyes, looks confused, and stares off blankly for several moments, in a fashion that reminds the doctor of a *petit mal* absence.[39] Slowly, Ms. Smith seems to return to awareness, and mumbles: "What were we talking about?" Dr. Hems' inquiry reveals that the patient is amnesic[40] for this strange incident, and efforts to explore it are to no avail.

As the Christmas holidays approach, Ms. Smith poignantly asks for a "big favor." Could she stay with Dr. Hems instead of visiting her insensitive parents?[41] She claims to be desperate, lonely, and panicked. Dr. Hems is torn; is this professional? Is it wise?[42] Her obvious vacillation creates a dramatic response in the patient: she is volcanically enraged. In scathing terms, Ms. Smith denounces Dr. Hems as "uncaring," " unfeeling," "sadistic," and "malevolent." She makes clear that the doctor's vicious refusal to grant such a modest request invalidates, in retrospect, the entire previous relationship, and calls into question the doctor's intentions, motivations, goodwill, and basic worth as a person.[43] Feeling ashamed and more than a little frightened, Dr. Hems acquiesces.[44]

Initially, things seem to quiet down, as Ms. Smith treats the house with a childlike wonder that charms Dr. Hems. All too soon, however, this period of calm is over, and the patient's demands again increase. Dr. Hems's already busy schedule begins to show serious work interference, and she finds herself torn between feelings of pity, rage and guilt. All urging by the doctor that her patient seek formal psychiatric help is met with enraged refusal at the implied abandonment.[45] Finally, Ms. Smith demands to be taken into bed by Dr. Hems and suckled at her breast like an infant; at this, the doctor finally draws the line.[46] Several hours are spent in convincing the patient to seek treatment. Finally, hospitalization is arranged and the exhausted physician gets some rest.

The hospital staff employ the "special care" and "understanding" originally recommended by Ms. Smith's internist—solidly buttressed, however, by firm and unequivocal attention to "limits."[47] After a transient flare-up, the patient, complaining bitterly about being neglected,[48] nevertheless appears to pull herself together and settle down to a more organized state. After a few weeks, she has returned to her job and is scheduled to engage in long-term outpatient treatment.[49]

Borderline Personality Disorder (BPD) end notes

1) "Lee" is an androgynous name. Patients with BPD may present as masculine women or as effeminate men, but are more likely to present in an undifferentiated, childlike manner. Most BPD patients are women. "Smith," the most common American name, conveys that patients with BPD may be found in all walks of life, from heroin-addicted street corner prostitutes to corporate Vice Presidents. BPD is an excellent illustration of the distinctions that can be drawn between illness (identified by diagnosis) and functioning.

2) Suicide attempts—particularly by overdose or transverse wrist cutting—are common paths for such patients to enter medical care. While some such attempts are serious and lethal, others are designed, not to die, but to live better, often by compelling others to respond in desired ways.

3) It is common for a flurry of communications, from both outside and inside the care setting, to precede such patients' arrival, an observation reflecting such patients' ability to mobilize concern.

4) The "non-maternal" parent is typically less involved with the patient. Note that the "maternal parent" may be a biological mother, adoptive parent, other relative, nanny, or anyone else who performs "mothering." This may also include fathers and other males.

5) This is the first time that the concept of "specialness" enters the case; it will not be the last.

6) BPD patients can mobilize great concern in others; contrast this with patients with schizophrenia, who may fade into the background, as it were.

7) Here, this particular minister-counselor stands in symbolically for the cohort of

partially trained treaters out there who may be in way over their heads with these difficult patients. This is not to suggest that such colleagues do not possess a unique skill set, or that they are not qualified to handle cases that comport with their own professionally defined competencies.

8) Why is the counselor so abusive to Dr. Hems, whom he has never even met? We can surmise that this anger is really about the patient, but instead is transferred onto the new doctor. Such "observer signs" prepare doctors for later conflicts among staff members on inpatient wards, where treater anger may be similarly misplaced. Cf. the Psychopathy vignette.

9) BPD patients may become "heavy users" of the medical system in order to fill their dependency needs. The non-specific symptoms noted here might be a contrivance for the patient to immerse herself in general medical care.

10) Dr. Hems is justifiably annoyed by the implicit suggestion that she need to be reminded to give "special care" to each of her patients. Patients with BPD may assume that they are not deemed worthy of care and that they must make special claims for it; here, the internist, having apparently bought into this assumption, is expressing that patient's worldview by proxy to Dr. Hems.

11) The specter of "specialness" looms again.

12) Here we see more use—and perhaps misuse or even abuse—of the medical system.

13) Such remarks are red flags, indicating the need for alertness to potential problems down the line.

14)   This case proffers one typical presentation of patients with BPD: a waif with a "tomboy" nuance and childlike demeanor. Other presentations might involve the tough, street-smart woman often seen in prison populations and the apparently normal woman whose psychopathology is initially masked.

15) BPD patients may look, speak, and dress younger than their stated age.

16) Obviously, this is guilt being used as a manipulative force.

17) Here is what psychiatrists call the "precipitant." Issues of separation are

very prominent in BPD and may trigger extreme reactions.

18) Dr. Hems does not simply usher the boyfriend out: she "finds herself" doing so, as

if she were an observer of an intention that emanates from outside herself. Treaters

may similarly find themselves in this position of enacting a patient's requests or

wishes, even against their own better judgment. Such personal "magnetism" of the

patient's wishes may lead to serious miscarriages of treatment.

19) Here is a direct, child-like appeal—unlike usual emergency room communications.

20) Clearly, at this point in her career (this is usually at around the seven-year mark)

Dr. Hems wants to improve her skills in attending to the psychology of ER patients.

Dr. Hems' readiness to listen and the patient's need to express produce an immediate

relational chemistry in this case.

21) There are many potential sources of romantic partnership problems for these

patients; the patient's neediness may be exhausting. Moreover, BPD women are

often searching for maternal-seeming boyfriends; not all boyfriends want to play

this role.

22) A family history of mental illness, not limited to BPD, is common, as is early

neglect or trauma.

23) Again, the non-maternal parent is more in the background; the intense feelings

focus on the maternal parent.

24) BPD is a disorder that may permit high work functioning; core problems arise in

the context of relationships.

25) Before the relationship with the treater intensifies, the patient's initial presentation is benign, even appealing.

26) Why is this detail relevant? BPD patients, having dealt with hard-to-read parents, have become nearly telepathic at reading treaters. A case on record describes a patient who realized the therapist was pregnant before the therapist realized this. We may assume that Ms. Smith picked up Dr. Hems' loneliness, at least subliminally, and responded to it.

27) For students in particular, such a suggestion of exclusive confiding would be highly seductive: that student is apparently being given a unique gift of information, separate from all those other professionals. In the present case, Dr. Hems is also taken with it.

28) This crucial comment heralds serious problems later on. On the surface, a compliment is ostensibly being paid to Dr. Hems, but it is in the form of a comparison. This is the thin end of an interpersonal wedge that will later become what psychiatrists call "splitting."

29) This is why Dr. Hems took that counseling course.

30)The first step on the downward road to perdition! Dr. Hems has bought into the subliminal theme of specialness and sees this patient as more special than that patient. Properly understood, that feeling could have alerted Dr. Hems and guided future interactions, but not here.

31) BPD patients may remain even in the most abusive or neglectful of relationships in order to meet dependency needs.

32) A common plea for more time with the doctor.

33) This example of setting a second appointment at the end of a full medical day captures the power and the intense "gravitational pull" of the patient's neediness.

34) This gratifying, positive feeling is regrettably only half of the curious defense mechanism of "splitting"—a means for the patient of affect management. Dr. Hems is "good" only insofar as someone else is "bad." (A medical student once referred to this as a "Jedi mind trick.")

35) Here is the "bad" side. Faced with managing both positive and negative feelings, sometimes toward the same person (ambivalence), BPD patients may allocate the positives to one person and the negatives to another, in order to tolerate both. This split often follows pre-existing divisions: therapist and prescriber; doctor and nurse; old staff and young staff; and medical student and resident.

36) As noted, the threat of separation may trigger extremely strong reactions. In addition, the sheer force of the boundless rage emanating from BPD patients may coerce even levelheaded treaters into caving in and altering their plans.

37) What is happening here is styled as "regression"—retreating, as an adaptive strategy, to the psychological and behavioral mechanisms of an earlier life stage; here, a more infantile, helpless one. When treaters provide limitless gratification without setting limits, this approach stirs up intense longings that overwhelm a patient's defenses and promote regression as a coping mechanism.

38) The presence of occasional frankly psychotic symptoms in patients with BPD caused lasting diagnostic and dynamic confusion; at one point such patients were referred to as having "pseudo-neurotic schizophrenia." Cooler heads prevailed: "micropsychoses," especially with paranoid trends, were seen as part of BPD symptomatology. The symptom here is an "illusion" —that is, a distortion of a real object, rather than a complete creation, as in hallucinations.

39) Such spontaneous trances are called "dissociation." Common forms are

fantasy, daydreaming, "highway hypnosis," and hypnosis itself. Patients with BPD may use this defense to deal with intense affect.

40) Amnesia for the dissociated event is common.

41) Again, Dr. Hems is "good," parents are "bad."

42) No.

43) Here, in the context of a perceived threatened rejection, the "split" is inverted: "good" becomes "bad," and vice versa. Remarkably, when in one side of a "split" state, the patient cannot recall ever having thought or felt the opposite.

44) Again, rage compels the target to acquiesce.

45) Even an appropriate referral feels like abandonment.

46) The natural end stage of an unchecked regression is infancy! (This vignette is based on a real case). The doctor draws the line none too soon.

47) The correct balance between gratifying and frustrating interactions is the art of therapy: too much gratification promotes regression, too much limit setting ("saying no") promotes flight from therapy. In general terms, treaters aim at gratifying adult, responsible strivings while rejecting infantile, regressive longings.

48) Such complaints often mark an appropriate balance: if the therapy is described as a bath of bliss, it usually means that someone else is getting the negatives.

49) In general, outpatient psychotherapy with adjunctive medications is the best approach. If hospitalization is necessary, it should be of short duration.

Psychopathy

When the phone rings, Dr. Hems mentally predicts that it will be another complaint from the nurses about Michael Scott[1], a patient on his neurology ward, where -- prior to Mr. Scott's arrival -- life used to proceed at a slow and measured pace, tinged with the aura of depression and futility common to neurology wards everywhere.

His prediction about the call confirmed, Dr. Hems gives the predictable curt response ("I'll talk to him about it") and hangs up[2]. Completing the predictability of this sequence, Dr. Hems' thoughts turn to a review of the case.

Mr. Scott is in his early thirties but already a pillar of his community[3]: owner of the largest local used-car dealership[4]; treasurer of his local Kiwanis chapter[5]; a regular church-goer[6]; and a close friend of many of the hospital's trustees[7]. This last distinction accounts, in fact, for his presence on Dr. Hems' ward. A trustee requested a "favor for a friend," that Dr. Hems take personal charge of Mr. Scott's case[8].

Mr. Scott's version of his history[9] was that he had been sitting in his car at a stoplight and had been hit by another car resulting in several injuries and persisting back pain, which had apparently been mishandled by other doctors[10]. Now, on the ward, a series of peculiar incidents has begun interrupting what Dr. Hems personally felt was a smooth hospital course. There was that time when a new nurse had sought out Dr. Hems in great distress, insisting she couldn't make sense out of what Mr. Scott was saying[11], when he exploded at her for keeping him waiting for his Percodan[12]. Then there was that time he blew up about being the last to

get served dinner one night…[13]

Shaking off this retrospective reverie, Dr. Hems soon arrives[14] on the ward and seeks out

Mr. Scott. The latter is sitting upright in bed[15], chatting amicably[16] with two giggling,

blushing[17] student nurses[18], who flee[19] as the doctor arrives. Wincing slightly[20], Mr. Scott

clambers out of bed to greet his doctor with a warm handclasp and sunny smile.[21] As usual,

Dr. Hems notes, not without a touch of envy, the patient's expensive bathrobe and impeccable

grooming[22].

As Mr. Scott stands, there is a dull click from the floor; both men look down and note a

yellow pill -- which Dr. Hems identifies as Valium -- wobbling toward the corner of the

room. Mr. Scott's eyes roll heavenward as Dr. Hems stoops for the pill:

"Jeez, that night nurse is a spastic!"[23] He elbows the doctor conspiratorially as his voice

lowers: "She drops pills, thermometers, bedpans — I think she's on the sauce![24] " He

winks knowingly. "Probably hides the bottle in the med cabinet next to the castor

oil![25,26] "

Dr. Hems cannot help smiling at this image, but he rearranges his face in serious lines

to report the nurses' complaint that Mr. Scott has been out of bed at night, disturbing other

patients and violating his "bed rest" prescription[27]. Mr. Scott's hands spread wide in a shrug

of helplessness.

"Doc! What am I gonna do? I tellya, I can't sleep with that old cancer fart snoring

in the next bed[28], the pain from my back is killing me, and the nurses" – his voice drops to a whisper as he leans closer [29] — "the nurses, I swear, they sit staring at my light on the board

and betting how long I can keep my thumb on the button! [30] They have a pool, see, and the

winner gets a pee bottle full of Johnny Walker. [31] "

Dr. Hems chuckles but has been distracted by a minty odor. "What's that smell?"

Mr. Scott smirks.

"I'm chewing a Breath-Saver. Makes me nice to be near, ya know? [32] " He turns serious:

"Look, Doc, I'm going home this week-end and I'll be away from work, taking it easy for a

coupla days; couldja gimme a script for that perky [33] stuff to cover the time? I'm running

kinda low."

Dr. Hems frowns. "Didn't I just last week— ["]

"Yeah, but my wife spilled some on the floor and I hadda throw them away."

Dr. Hems looks thoughtful. "I don't have my pad with me; maybe the nursing

station--"

Mr. Scott holds up a hasty hand: "Hey, no sweat, Doc; you can use my notepaper

here."

Dr. Hems looks dubious. Mr. Scott's wink conveys: "Leave it to me."

"It's okay, Doc, I been doin' business with this pharmacy for years; you could write it

on toilet paper [34] and they'd still cash it -uh, fill it, I mean. [35] "

"All right. "Dr. Hems scrawls hastily, then prepares to depart. "I'll talk to the nurses

about –" [36]

Mr. Scott's gratitude is profound:

"Hey, I'd really appreciate that, Doc; sometimes I think you're my only friend. [37] "

He claps Dr. Hems on the back. Dr. Hems, who would feel annoyed at this liberty from any other patient, experiences an inexplicable warm glow [38] that lingers as he starts

down the hall [39]. Three strides out of the door he remembers that he had planned to ask Mr.

Scott about the balance due on his bill for office visits last month [40], but he mentally

dismisses the impulse as something he can take care of later.

The nursing station radiates suppressed tension as Dr. Hems enters. Ms. Anderson, the

most senior nurse, clears her throat with the air of speaking for the group.

"If I may ask, Doctor, how long will Mr. Scott be --ah –recuperating with us? [41] "

Dr. Hems' anger flares. [42]

"As long as I feel it is indicated!" he snarls. "And another thing, Mrs. Anderson: he's

a paying patient here and entitled to adequate nursing services! [43] I'm getting tired of this

incessant griping and I want it to stop!"

As Dr. Hems storms out, to the sound of gasps of outrage, an unoccupied part of his

mind is musing that he has called Mrs. Anderson "Katie" for the last eleven years. [44]

Psychopathy endnotes

1) Scott, as in "scot-free." Unsuccessful or maladroit psychopaths are often caught by the criminal justice system. Successful psychopaths like this one may go scot-free and rise to positions of authority, holding political office, becoming CEOs of large corporations and playing other similar roles. In contrast, the official criteria of the diagnosis of "anti-social personality disorder" consist of a list of failures: school, work, legal trouble, relationships and so on; that diagnosis suits criminals and the inmates of the prison system. Confusingly, the term "sociopath" is used in some contexts as a simple synonym for psychopath, but in other settings it refers to perpetrators of serial sexual homicide. You have to ask.

2) Note for clarity that Dr. Hems has agreed to confront Mr. Scott on behalf of the nurses; it would be useful to remember this.

3) To be a pillar of the community requires a number of adaptive traits: charisma, financial success, being a "people person", showing leadership, involving others and having an unblemished record.

4) Stereotypes aside, a successful dealer must rapidly assess new customers coming in -- from haircut to shoes -- and must efficiently direct them, without wasting time, to a car that will be likely to appeal. In contrast to what occurs with other mental illnesses, symptomatic distortions do not interfere with this procedure for the psychopath, who may be highly skilled at reading others.

5) History tells us that any fool can be vice president; but to be chosen treasurer of your lodge signifies the ability to inspire trust.

6) Going regularly to church is merely behavior: it does not distinguish between the devout believer and the someone who is merely observing social convention. Unlike the patient with schizophrenia, who may be deaf to social cues, the psychopath can tune in

to such signals successfully. In some communities one could not be considered a pillar without regular and visible church attendance. More broadly, because of such ordinary behaviors, the differential diagnosis for "psychopath" includes "normal."

7) This may represent "all of the above."

8) This kind of arrangement may induce "VIP Syndrome," where the patient admitted in this manner may feel entitled to special treatment, and the case may be "run from the top" rather than by front-line clinicians.

9) But isn't every history the patient's version?

10) An assertion of past mishandling is usually a red flag for trouble.

11) This reaction is less likely for Mr. Scott, but some psychopaths decompensate when locked in for the night or thwarted in some other way; under stress such patients may briefly resemble persons with paranoid schizophrenia.

12) To fill an inner void, psychopaths may rely on substance abuse and exhibit drug seeking behaviors. Others fill the void by risk-taking and other dangerous behavior, in order to feel at least something.

13) One index of "VIP syndrome" is narcissistic entitlement: "Someone needs to be last to get served dinner, but it won't be me!" A variant sign is victim entitlement:" I have suffered so much [in this case, back pain], that you owe me."

14) Going onto your ward quietly, without fuss or ceremony, is an excellent way for physicians to observe unexpected things, as now happens to Dr. Hems in the following scene.

15) Sitting upright in bed actually aggravates legitimate back pain.

16) Amicability is rare in hospitalized pain patients.

17) Giggling alone could result from mere banter or joking; blushing, however, reveals, via the autonomic nervous system, that Mr. Scott has been flirting.

18) Because of their lack of advanced training and experience and perhaps with present

naïveté as well, the student nurses are the most vulnerable persons on a ward; staff in their position may be preferentially "targeted."

19) The students do not leave: they "flee." This manner of departure conveys that they feel guilty of having been temporarily de-professionalized. Nurses have a professional code that they try not to violate; the patient has no such code and may act without constraint.

20) Now that the doctor has arrived, wincing sets in.

21) Handclasp and smile are essential to sales success; unlike the psychopath, persons with other illnesses (schizophrenia, depression) may not typically respond in this fashion.

22) Envy of patients is a rarely discussed phenomenon that may impair objectivity when treating celebrities, local dignitaries or other VIPs. The conventional wisdom regarding physicians suggests that they deal with their own dependency needs by taking care of others and then identifying with the recipients of that care -- an identification that can slide over into envy.

23, 24) This is a critical moment: Mr. Scott seems to have been caught red-handed while hoarding a controlled substance. But does he blush, stammer, or act baffled by how that pill got there? He does not. Without hesitation, he smoothly shifts the blame to another, provides a possible motive for that other's conduct, and goes scot-free. Some authorities note that psychopaths have decreased autonomic reactivity: they rarely blush, sweat or stammer when confronted; this advantage often enables them to pass casual and formal tests of deception.

25, 26) Elbowing and winking invite Dr. Hems to enter into Mr. Scott's view of the situation. This is a narcissistic seduction: not about sex but about self-esteem: a VIP is including Dr. Hems into the inner circle by confiding in him, up close and personal; the phenomenon is analogous to telling a used car customer what a terrific bargain he is getting. In addition, Dr. Hems is invited to ally with Mr. Scott against the nurse; this kind of misalliance is termed "splitting": breaking team unity by pitting one team member against another. Importantly, this feat is accomplished purely non-verbally, by physical actions; had Dr. Hems been invited verbally to decide whom he believed, patient or nurse, he would likely hesitate out of suspicion.

27) This is what Dr. Hems came for, as requested by the nurses. Mission accomplished?

28) When directly confronted, under pressure, Mr. Scott's lack of empathy breaks out via this crude and unfeeling expression. Psychopaths often have their empathic capacity beaten or neglected out of them in childhood, facilitating their exploitation of others, and leading – in more extreme instances – to violence, torture and murder. In contrast, ordinary persons may be constrained by their empathic engagement with a potential victim.

29) Leaning in and lowering his voice reestablishes the misalliance and narcissistic seduction by means of physical action.

30) This is a classic example of psychopathic truth: it is <u>somewhat</u> true but omits a critical point, usually involving personal responsibility: we can infer that Mr. Entitlement has hit that button so often the nurses are understandably reluctant to respond quickly. This also creates a de- professionalizing impact, since nurses are in fact supposed to respond. A psychopath on death row for murder once explained his situation as: "The knife just went in." This was true – but, of course, incomplete.

31) Note that Mr. Scott, in a conversation that has nothing to do with alcohol, alludes to it twice as a factor; such preoccupation may be a clue to the most under-diagnosed disorder in medicine: alcoholism.

32) …And hides the smell of alcohol as well.

33) A patient may try to disguise overt drug seeking by pretending to be confused about the exact name of the substance being sought.

34) This sounds strange and hyperbolic, but since it is <u>psychopathic</u> truth, it may be true; the missing element may be that some illegal activity is going on with this pharmacy.

35) A Freudian slip? A hint that some check forgery may also be involved? We'll never know.

36) Wait -- what? Dr. Hems is going to confront the nurses on behalf of Mr. Scott? But did

he not come for the exact opposite purpose, to confront Mr. Scott on behalf of the nurses? To follow this process, note the preceding dialogue, in which Dr. Hems does not get to finish a sentence before Mr. Scott has grasped the expected end of the sentence and supplied an answer and an alibi. Arguably, in this brief conversation, Mr. Scott is thinking faster and perhaps better than Dr. Hems; we may contrast this with the disabling thought disturbances seen in other mental disorders.

37) A direct pitch to Dr. Hems' self esteem.

38) If there has, indeed, been a narcissistic seduction, then that glow is orgasm: Dr. Hems feels approved of by a pillar of the community.

39) Just like the feeling of having gotten a good deal -- for example, a special bargain on a car.

40) Psychopaths may not take financial responsibilities all that seriously.

41) As opposed to simple "recuperating," "ah—recuperating" is shorthand for: "This patient is treating this like a hotel, I'm not even sure he's really sick, and I want him off my ward."

42) The result of such splitting is that treatment team members wind up fighting with one another.

43) Resorting to the official policies at a time like this is a proven recipe for failed communication.

44) The regrettable success of such splitting is to drive a wedge between the principals in this highly significant, long-standing professional relationship. Medical interns are warned that a good relationship with the senior nurse is the single most determinative factor in whether they will ever get any sleep at night.

Suggested readings

1) Black DW, Andreasen NC: Introductory textbook of psychiatry, 6th ed. American Psychiatric Publishing, 2014

2) Sadock BJ, Sadock VA: Kaplan and Sadock's Concise textbook of psychiatry, 3rd ed., Lippincott Williams and Wilkins, 2008

3) Cutler J: Psychiatry. Oxford University Press, 2014

4) Hales RE, Yudofsky SC: American Psychiatric Publishing Textbook of psychiatry. American Psychiatric Publishing, 2008